Run For Your Life

How to Start a Habit that Last

Effendy Hu

ISBN: 9798883612151

DEDICATION

To my beloved wife, kids and family especially my mom, thank you for always being by my side. You have been my rock through the highs and lows of life and I couldn't be more grateful for your unconditional love and support. You have been my biggest cheerleaders and have believed in me when I didn't believe in myself. I'm so lucky to have such an incredible group of people in my life and I wouldn't be the same without you all.

CONTENTS

ACKNOWLEDGMENTS

I would like to express my deepest gratitude to my mentors, who has been a constant source of guidance, support and encouragement throughout my journey. Your wisdom and experience have been invaluable to me and I am truly grateful for the time you have invested in me. Thank you for believing in me.

I would also like to thank my teachers, for providing a solid foundation in learning and for inspiring me to pursue my passions.

I am also grateful to my friends and family for their love and support. Their unwavering belief in me and encouragement have been a source of strength and motivation.

Finally, I would like to thank each and every person who has contributed, directly or indirectly, to my success. Your contributions have been instrumental in helping me reach this milestone. Thank you all for being a part of my life.

1 START WITH A WHY

If I had a DeLorean and went back 20 years to tell my younger self that in the future I would run daily, my younger self wouldn't have believed a single word of it. Growing up in Indonesia, I was never a sporty person. I had no interest in sports whatsoever. I recall my secondary school days, where the prospect of PE lessons filled me with dread. One vivid memory stands out—during a PE assessment that required us to run a cross-country race, I was convinced I might collapse from exhaustion. Anticipating stitches, cramps, and soreness, I dreaded the ordeal.

Fast forward to when my son was in primary school, around grade 3 or 4. After his cross-country run, he excitedly shared that he had come second to last in the class. In that moment, I knew that I need to do something. I felt compelled to take action, to spare my son from the same disappointment I had experienced in my own childhood.

This became my 'why' when I embarked on my journey of running, and I urge you to discover your own 'why' as well. Having a purpose makes establishing the habit much easier. It serves as motivation during challenging times and when enthusiasm wanes. Your 'why' is a constant reminder of a higher purpose, transcending the mere act of running.

Your 'why' should resonate emotionally; without that connection, it may not endure as long as one rooted in genuine emotion.

Day 1 Exercise:
Spend some time writing your 'why'; reflect on what this newfound commitment to running signifies for you. Why is it important? Is it to train someone else, like me, or do you aim to embrace a more active and

healthier lifestyle? Consider the deeper reasons behind your decision. Treat this seriously as a contract to yourself; it is a promise to hold yourself accountable. Once you have written your journal, take the time to read it back to yourself. Do you feel any emotion? Does it move you? Does it sound convincing? If your friends or family members were to read this journal, would they believe it? Document these reflections in your journal so that you can easily refer back to them during challenging times.

You can write down your why below, when you write it down, there it helps you being accountable to yourself.

....

....

....

....

....

....

....

If you are brave enough you can announce it to the world through social media, so that everyone can hold you accountable. When you have others holding you accountable, you are most likely to follow through.

2 HABIT FORMATION

Now that you have your strong 'why,' it is time to cultivate the habit to achieve your running goals. According to Charles Duhigg, the author of 'The Power of Habit,' there is a specific pattern to follow to initiate a new habit and ensure its persistence. Once it becomes a habit, you won't need to think much about it—similar to the routine of brushing your teeth in the morning and evening.

So, how do you establish this habit loop? It goes like this: **Trigger - Action - Reward - Repeat**. You need to set this habit loop to ensure it sticks. For example, if your current trigger after dinner is seeing the remote on the couch, and you reach for it to flip channels or start Netflix, the next thing you know, you're engrossed in a show until late at night. This pattern repeats itself, becoming part of your evening routine.

Let's break down this event: the *trigger* is seeing the remote on the couch, the *action* is watching Netflix, and the *reward* is feeling good about spending time enjoying the movie. This pattern *repeats* the following day and subsequent days.

Now, if you want to establish a new running habit, you'll need the same habit loop. Set up your *trigger*—perhaps placing your running shoes next to your bed or hanging your favourite exercise outfit where it's the first thing you see upon waking up.

Next, engage in the *action* of running. Start small—500 meters or just around the smallest block near your house. It only takes 5 minutes.

Follow this with a strong *reward* after the run to reinforce the action. This could be a coffee around the corner, a big breakfast waiting for you, a croissant, a donut, KFC or any indulgence you fancy.

Ensure you can repeat this pattern—trigger-action-reward—for the next 7 weeks for it to register as a habit. It might be tempting to break the routine halfway, but sticking to it is crucial; otherwise, you'll need to reset and start again. Not even once should you deviate to ensure the habit sticks. Once it becomes ingrained, you can take a break once or twice (never more than twice), knowing you'll easily get back into it the following day.

For me, my trigger is simply waking up; I don't have a physical cue. My reward is a satisfying big breakfast after the run.

Day 2 Exercise:

Set up your running habit pattern and commit to it for at least 7 weeks. While it's not mandatory to run every day, the habit will form more rapidly if you do so. Alternatively, establish a routine for three times or twice a week. Ensure you have also defined a consistent reward after each run to complete the loop. It needs to be consistent and reliable; mark it in your calendar or diary, and stick to it for the full 7 weeks.

Do not skip this exercise and refrain from progressing to the next chapter until you have completed it.

You can use the following running tracker to track your activity, the idea is to mark each day that you are running, and make sure that you didn't break the chain of crosses

Running Tracker

WEEK	SUN	MON	TUE	WED	THU	FRI	SAT
1							
2							
3							
4							
5							
6							
7							

3 WHAT GETS MEASURED GETS IMPROVED

Peter Drucker, a legendary management consultant quoted in his book "The Effective Executive," said, "What is measured, improves." You might be wondering what this has to do with running. In today's age, where many of us seek instant gratification, it can be challenging to wait for results.

Enter the device to track your run. You don't have to own an expensive "Apple Watch," "Galaxy Watch," "Fitbit," or any tracker for that matter. You might already have one, so why not use it? If you don't already own any of these devices, you can use your phone to track. Whether you're an Apple or Android person, your phone likely has an app that tracks your movement or exercise.

All you need to do is bring it with you during your run; it will automatically track how long you've been running and may provide statistics on calories burned, heart rate, etc. For more precise measurements, you can invest in one of the fitness devices mentioned above. Personally, I don't use any device, but I always track my progress through the "Strava" app for the reasons mentioned earlier. I like to know my run's speed and duration, as it helps me understand how to improve my speed, distance, or duration. Plus, who doesn't love a bit of healthy competition for bragging rights?

If you would like to follow me on Strava, here is the link:
https://www.strava.com/athletes/effendyhu

Day 3 Exercise:

You can either use a fitness device to track your run or simply use your phone; the choice is yours. Make sure you track your progress every time you go for a run, even for a simple jog. There's something satisfying about completing your run, which will keep you motivated. Feeling good about your progress makes habit formation much easier because it encourages you to do it more.

Wouldn't it feel good when you can see your progression charts similar to the one below?

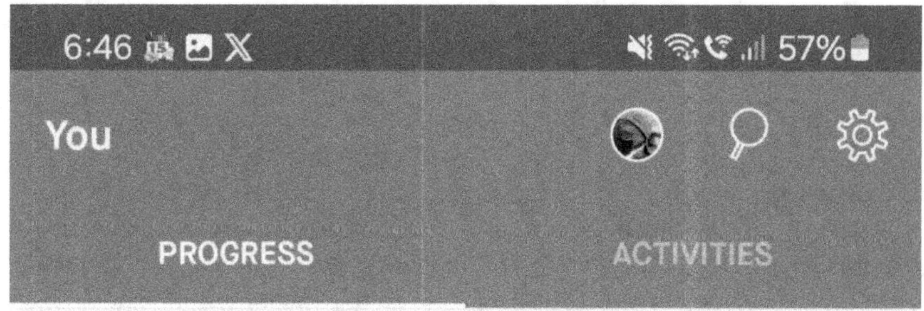

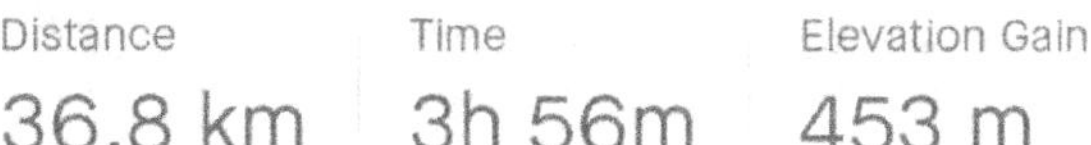

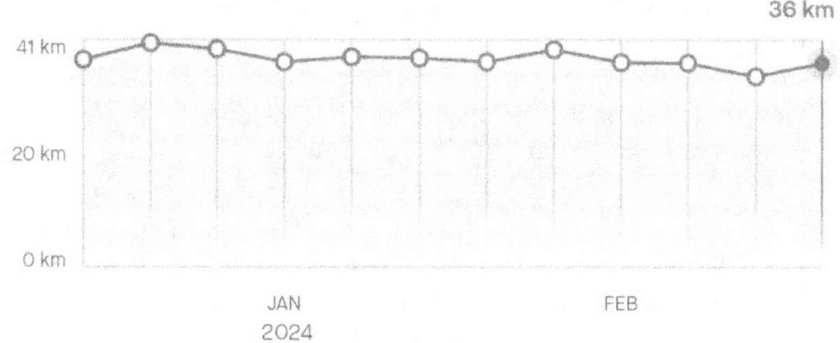

3 TIME MANAGEMENT

When it comes to exercise, people often claim they don't have time. They express a wish to find the time to squeeze it into their busy schedules. In reality, these statements are often excuses, indicating that exercise is not currently a priority for them. The truth is, if you genuinely want to do something, you will make the time for it, especially for activities you are passionate about. For instance, you rarely hear people saying they don't have time to watch a movie they like; instead, they plan their life and schedules around it.

If you don't allocate time for exercise now, you may find yourself having to make time for illness or medical procedures later on in life – that's how it works. Let that sink in for a minute.

So, how can you find the time? It's simple: identify the most convenient time for your running and plan or integrate your daily activities around it. This could be in the early morning, on the way to work, while dropping your kids off at school, during lunchtime, when picking up your kids from school, upon returning from work, or any time that suits you.

If you still can't seem to find a suitable time, consider waking up 30 minutes earlier to make room for it. If you look hard enough, you'll likely discover a slot that fits your schedule. If you genuinely can't find the time, then perhaps this book may not be the right fit for you.

Day 3 Exercise:
Retrieve your calendar, whether it's an online platform or paper-based, and identify the most convenient 30-minute slot in your day. Schedule this as a recurring meeting, so it's consistently reserved, requiring no additional

thought. If scheduling the same time every day proves challenging, that's okay; you can vary the time depending on the day. The key is to establish the habit and eliminate an extra thing to remember.

If you're not accustomed to using a calendar for your day-to-day activities, now might be an excellent time to cultivate that habit too. Personally, I use Google Calendar and share it with my wife, ensuring we operate with a unified family calendar. Since adopting this approach, we've experienced no issues with double bookings or confusion about wshere we are supposed to be or where our kids' activities are.

4 BREATHING EXERCISE

You might be wondering why you need to learn how to breathe, given that you've been doing it throughout your life. Indeed, up until now, you've been breathing sufficiently to supply oxygen to your lungs, supporting your body's basic functions. However, what I'm about to teach you is a technique that goes beyond basic breathing. It's a method designed to prime your body, providing the stamina necessary not only for running but also for various other activities you enjoy.

One such exercise is called "box breathing," where you inhale for a count of four, hold your breath for a count of four, exhale for a count of four, and hold your breath for a count of four. Repeat this exercise several times to help calm your mind and regulate your breathing.

Another useful exercise is "breath control," where you focus on controlling the length and depth of your inhales and exhales. Start by inhaling deeply for a count of four, then exhale slowly for a count of six. Gradually increase the length of your exhale until it is twice as long as your inhale. This exercise can help you become more aware of your breathing and build up your endurance.

The one I wanted to cover in detail is "Wim Hof" breathing technique. The Wim Hof breathing technique is a powerful method that can help improve our overall health and wellbeing. This technique, named after its creator Wim Hof, is a combination of deep breathing exercises and meditation. One of the main benefits of this technique is that it can help you hold your breath for longer periods of time. By increasing the oxygen levels in your body, you can improve your lung capacity and enhance your overall physical and mental performance. This technique has been clinically proven to yield health benefits. Personally, I can attest to its efficacy as I've been able to increase my body temperature on cold winter nights through the consistent practice of this breathing technique.

Overall, practicing the Wim Hof breathing technique can provide numerous benefits, including increased lung capacity, reduced stress and anxiety levels, and improved overall physical and mental performance.

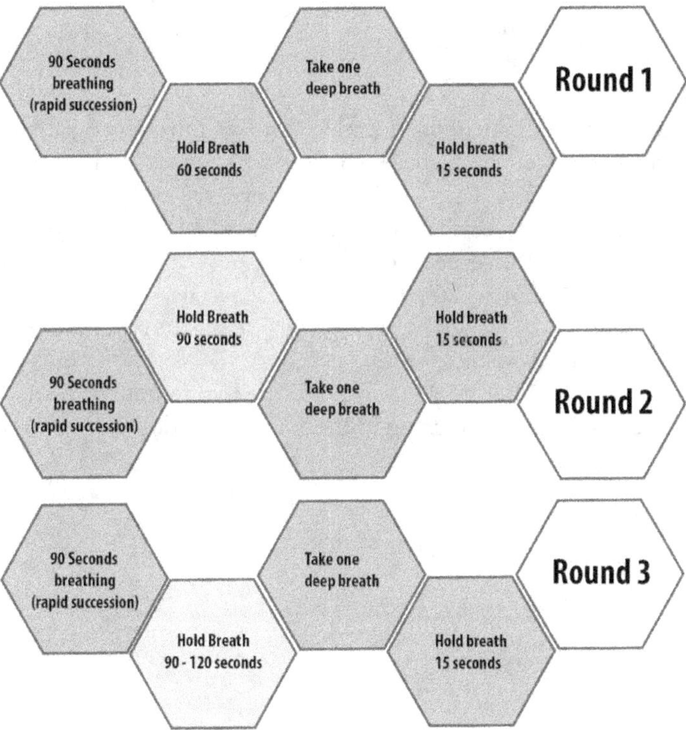

The breathing method that I am going to introduce to you consists of the 3 rounds, it will take approximately 15 minutes to complete. This exercise needs to be done while you are sitting or lying down on a bed. You don't want to do this exercise while standing up of doing chores, as you might collapse.

-   The first round consists of the breathing in and out in rapid succession for the 90 seconds, followed by holding your breath for approximately 60 seconds, and then taking one big inhale and hold your breath again for 15 seconds before exhaling. Then, immediately move on to the second round,
-   Second round starts with breathing in and out again in rapid

succession for the 90 seconds, followed by holding your breath for as long as you can, in this second round you should aim to exceed the length of the first round, aim for 90 seconds. After that, take one big inhale and hold your breath again for 15 seconds before exhaling.
- Finally, continue on to the last round with rapid succession of breathing for another 90 seconds, followed by breath holding for approximately one to two minutes before taking a big inhale and holding your breath again for 15 seconds. Then, continue with breathing normally.

Day 4 Exercise:
Practice the Wim Hof breathing exercise that was introduced earlier. Find a comfortable and quiet place to lie down, such as your bed, to allow your body and mind to relax. This will help you preserve oxygen and hold your breath longer. The aim of the exercise is to gradually stretch your breath-holding capacity. If you're new to this exercise, start with 30 seconds and work your way up to one minute, and eventually two minutes. Be patient and allow your body to adjust, clear your mind and relax to help you achieve longer breath-holding times.
It will take some time before you can reach the two minutes pause.
You can use the Guided breathing in the following video link
https://www.youtube.com/watch?v=0BNejY1e9ik&t=2s

5 UPHILL BATTLE

I'm sure you've run in the past, and this might not be your first time lacing up your running shoes. However, your past experiences may not have been as comfortable as you'd like, and that's likely why you've turned to this book. At this point, I encourage you to forget everything you think you know about running. Approach this with a fresh start and an open mind. This mindset will be crucial when faced with challenges, as it's essential to stay true to your 'why.' Without a strong 'why,' the temptation to give up when things get tough becomes more significant. If you're struggling to find your 'why,' consider revisiting the exercise from Chapter 1. You did complete the exercise, didn't you?

Stick to your schedule, at least for the initial 7 weeks, to cement those habits. Begin with a modest distance, perhaps just 500m around the block, to keep the momentum going. The actual distance isn't crucial at this point; the key is to maintain the habit and make it stick. As you develop more stamina and strength, you can gradually increase the distance.

The exercises from the previous chapter should have contributed to building your stamina, allowing you to establish a regular breathing pattern aligned with your running pace – breathing in through your nose and out through your mouth.

In this chapter, I also want to emphasise the importance of your body posture while running. This is crucial for minimizing the impact and reducing the risk of injury. Running in the right posture can make a significant difference in your overall experience.

Here's a guide to ensure you maintain the correct form:

1. **Head and Eyes**: Keep your head upright and eyes looking straight ahead. Avoid tilting your head up or down.
2. **Shoulders:** Relax your shoulders and keep them squared, avoiding tension. Let your arms hang naturally by your sides.
3. **Arms**: Maintain a 90-degree angle at your elbows, with your arms swinging forward and backward in a relaxed motion. Avoid crossing your arms in front of your body.
4. **Hands at your Waist**: Keep your hands relaxed, with a light fist or an open palm. Avoid clenching your fists, as tension can travel up your arms.
5. **Torso and Back**: Keep your torso upright and engage your core muscles. Avoid leaning forward or backward, as this can strain your back.
6. **Hips**: Keep your hips in a neutral position, avoiding excessive tilting forward or backward.
7. **Legs and Stride**: Take short, quick steps with your feet landing directly beneath your hips. Avoid overstriding, as this can lead to discomfort and potential injury.
8. **Feet**: Land on your midfoot, ensuring a soft and controlled landing. Avoid heavy heel-striking, as this can cause excess impact on your joints.

By maintaining this proper running posture, you'll enhance your running efficiency, reduce the risk of injury, and contribute to an overall more enjoyable running experience.

Cadence refers to the number of steps you take per minute while running. Increasing your cadence can help reduce the impact on your body and minimize the risk of injury. Strive for a cadence of around 180 steps per minute, though individual variations may apply. To improve your cadence, focus on shortening your stride and taking quicker, lighter steps.

The way you land and push off the ground can significantly impact the forces transmitted through your body. Here are some tips for an optimal landing and push-off technique:
   a. Landing: Aim for a soft, controlled landing with your foot underneath your body. Avoid landing on your heels, as it can increase the impact and strain on your joints. Instead, focus on a midfoot strike, where your foot makes initial contact with the ground.
   b. Push-off: As your foot leaves the ground, focus on propelling

yourself forward using the muscles in your legs and hips. Imagine pushing off the ground with your toes, which can help engage the powerful muscles in your posterior chain (calves, hamstrings, and glutes).

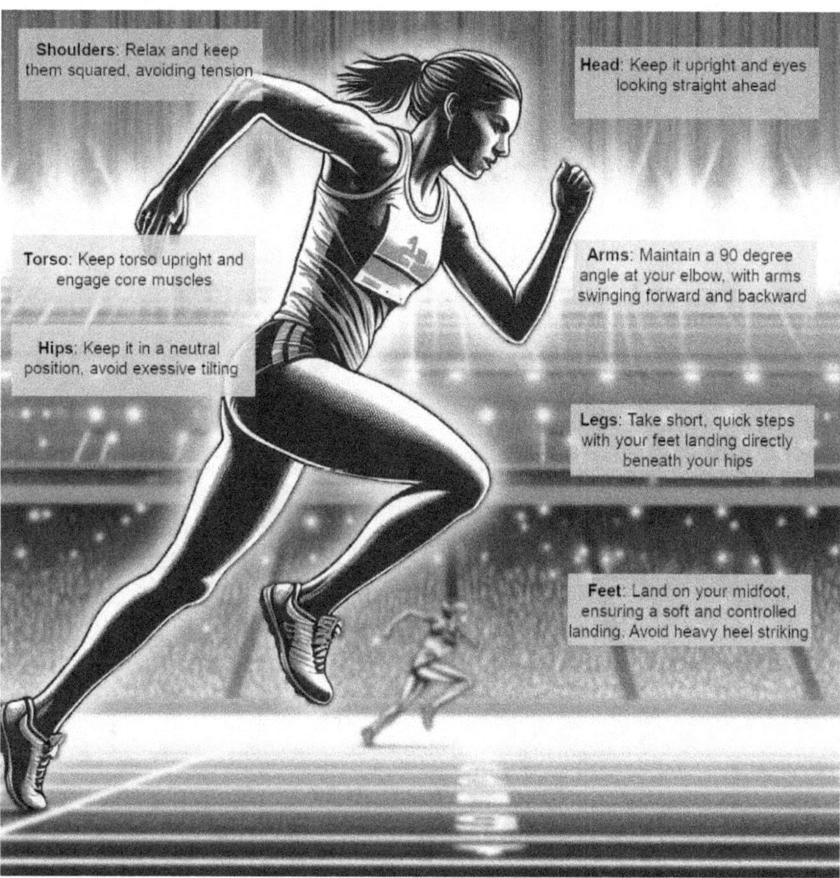

While proper running posture is essential for reducing the risk of injury, it's equally important to allow your body to adapt gradually to the demands of running. Increase your mileage and intensity gradually, allowing your muscles, bones, and connective tissues to strengthen and adapt. Listen to your body, and if you experience persistent pain or discomfort, consult a healthcare professional or a running specialist.

Day 5 Exercise:
Begin your running routine according to the schedule you've set up. The key is consistency; it's better to start small than not start at all. I understand that life will inevitably present obstacles, and you'll find a myriad of reasons

why you can't run on a particular day. However, the real reason is not lack of time; it's a matter of not prioritising your commitment to running. Rather than making excuses, remember your strong 'why,' stick to your schedule to establish the habit, and avoid making excuses.

Lastly, repeat day 3 exercise to keep track of your progress. If you don't have a smartwatch or Fitbit, that's okay—simply use your mobile phone.

Remember, what gets tracked also gets improved. Utilise this tool to reinforce your habit formation and complete the habit loop.

6 WHAT'S NEXT

Now that you have established your daily running habits and are tracking your progress, it's time to take it to the next level. Here are some suggestions on what that next level might entail. By all means, this is not an exhaustive list. While many of the following events are in Melbourne, Australia, you can likely find similar events in your area. If not, perhaps you can take the initiative and champion the start of such events yourself.

-   Run **"The Tan"** (**3.8** km): If you are in Melbourne, Australia, head to the Botanical Gardens in the city and join the active community running during their lunch breaks or participating in fundraising events. For more information, visit their website at https://runthetan.net/about-us/

-   Run for the Kids event (short course **4.6** km, long course **14.5** km): Another popular run for charity event in Melbourne, Australia. Learn more at https://www.runforthekids.com.au/

-   Run a half marathon (**21.1** km): Melbourne, Australia hosts a half marathon event. Details can be found at https://melbournemarathon.com.au/events/

-   Run a full marathon (**42.2** km).

-   Participate in the World Virtual Ekiden run: Ekiden is a relay run popular in Japan, with professional runners making a career out of it. Distances vary; for example, the Mount Fuji Ekiden covers 47 kilometers (29 miles), while the Grand Tour Kyushu spans 739 kilometers (458 miles). Although daunting, these distances are divided among multiple runners on each team. You may only run a 5K leg, as former professional runner Katie Newton did when she participated in the Chiba Ekiden for the U.S. team.

- Consider completing a mini Triathlon if it's on your bucket list. Swimming is a prerequisite for this, and if you're interested in learning how to swim, I've written a book on mastering this skill in 30 days. I myself learned to swim as an adult, so it's definitely achievable and may one day save your life.

Day 6 Exercise:
Participate in one of the events mentioned above. You'll earn exclusive bragging rights and feel good knowing you're supporting a charitable cause. Crossing the finish line will also bring a sense of personal achievement.

Congratulations on completing your 6-day exercise challenge to keep you on the healthy track. You should give yourself a pat on the back. Celebrate the achievement and continue repeating the habit loop for 7 weeks.

BONUS CHAPTER - QUICK FIRE VISUALISATION

Recently, I read a book about manifesting dreams through mental exercise using a technique called quick-fire visualization. I believe this exercise could be beneficial for achieving your goal, particularly in establishing the running habit. Approach this exercise with intention and focus; you may find it helpful to have a cup of tea to clear your mind.

Here are the steps:

1. Visualize the desired event, as if watching it on TV. For instance, imagine running a marathon. Picture what you see, feel, and smell in the air.
2. Shrink the image and turn it black and white.
3. Step outside of yourself, observing as if experiencing an out-of-body moment, watching yourself watch the TV.
4. Rewind the 'movie' just before the perfect moment. Then fast-forward, transitioning into the future. Turn the scene into color and 3D, immersing yourself in the sounds of success.
5. When you reach a feeling of 10 out of 10, snap your fingers to anchor that sensation.
6. Rapidly rewind the 'movie' to find that happy feeling again, and snap your fingers to anchor another sensation.
7. Step into the TV and visualize yourself doing everything necessary to achieve your goal.
8. Amplify the feeling's volume until reaching level 10, then snap your fingers.
9. Repeat the process of rewinding and fast-forwarding, snapping your fingers at each happy ending.

Turn this exercise into a daily habit, incorporating it into your routine.
I wish you success in establishing the running habit and achieving a healthy, happy life.

Thank you for completing this book; it marks the first step in your habit formation journey."

ABOUT THE AUTHOR

Effendy was born overseas and migrated to Australia in his late twenties. He didn't do much exercise back in Indonesia as that was not his priority back then.

These days, Effendy is an avid fitness enthusiast who maintains a healthy lifestyle. He starts his day with a daily 5 km run followed by cold showers, and regularly attends swimming sessions at his local pool to maintain his swimming skills.

Effendy hopes to continue to inspire others to take up running or exercise and embrace a healthy lifestyle.

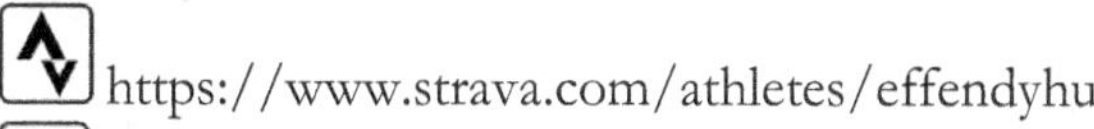 https://www.strava.com/athletes/effendyhu

@effendyhu

https://www.instagram.com/effendypin/